D1451308

CONSUMERS' GUIDE TO
Top Doctors

BY THE EDITORS OF CONSUMERS' CHECKBOOK MAGAZINE

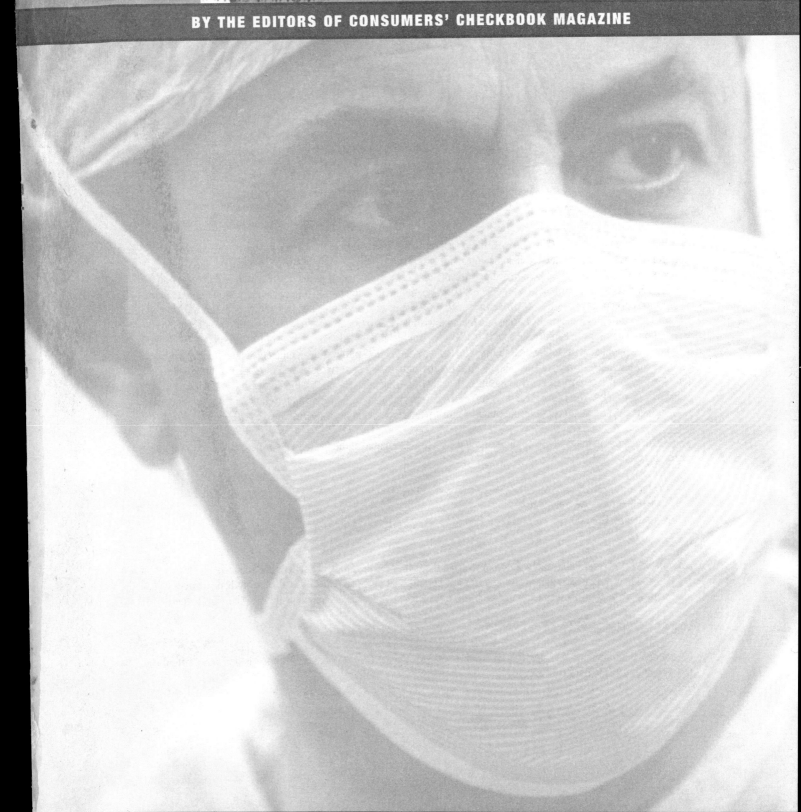

This book is a publication of Consumers' CHECKBOOK, which is a program of the Center for the Study of Services, a nonprofit organization dedicated to helping consumers find high-quality, reasonably priced service providers and retailers. Founded in 1974, the Center is supported by sales of its publications and other research and information products and services, in print and on the Web, and by tax-deductible donations from consumers. None of the Center's publications accept any advertising. *Consumers' CHECKBOOK* magazines, published by the Center in the Washington, DC, area and the San Francisco Bay Area, rate the quality and prices of local service firms of various kinds, ranging from auto repair shops to banks to hospitals. The Center will be launching local versions of *Consumers' CHECKBOOK* in other metropolitan areas in the near future. The Center's *BARGAINS* publications guide consumers to low-priced retailers for big-ticket products. The Center's CarBargains and LeaseWise services assist consumers in finding the lowest available prices for new car purchasing or leasing by having new car dealers bid competitively for the consumer's business. The Center also does survey, research, and analysis activities under contract with government agencies, employer coalitions, nonprofit public sector organizations, and health plans.

More information on the Center's publications and services is available at the Center's Web site, *www.checkbook.org* or by contacting us at:

Center for the Study of Services
733 15th Street, NW, Suite 820
Washington, DC 20005
202-347-7283

No commercial use: Publications and reports from the Center for the Study of Services are solely for the use of their readers and may not be used in advertising or for any commercial purpose. The Center for the Study of Services will take steps to prevent or prosecute commercial uses of excerpted materials, its name, or the *CHECKBOOK* name.